Consultations & Appointments Form Organiser for Holistic Nutrition Therapists

by G St George

All Rights Reserved. No part of this publication may be reproduced in any form or by any means, including scanning, photocopying, or otherwise without prior written permission of the copyright holder. Copyright © 2019

Therapist name ....

Address..

....

Telephone number................................

Appointments

Name	Phone number, email address	Date/Time	Notes

Appointments

Name	Phone number, email address	Date/Time	Notes

Appointments

Name	Phone number, Email address	Date/Time	Notes

Appointments

Name	Phone number, email address	Date/Time	Notes

Appointments

Name	Phone number, email address	Date/Time	Notes

Appointments

Name	Phone number, email address	Date/Time	Notes

Appointments

Name	Phone number, email address	Date/Time	Notes

HOLISTIC NUTRITION CONSULTATION FORM

Therapist:	Clinic:	Date:
Client's name:	Age:	Gender:
Height	Weight	BMI
Client' address: Tel No:	Occupation:	Doctor's address/ telephone no.

CLIENT'S HEALTH OBJECTIVES

WHAT HEALTH ISSUES & SYMPTOMS CONCERN THE CLIENT?

TYPICAL FOODS & DRINKS CONSUMED DURING THE DAY + QUANTITIES

Breakfast	Lunch
Dinner	Snacks between meals
Fruit & vegetables	Water

Other drinks	Supplements (if any)

DIGESTION & ELIMINATION

Slow digestion	Acid reflux	Indigestion	Stomach pain
Bloating	IBS	Wind	Nausea after eating
Stool type & frequency	Undigested food in stool	Pain anywhere else in the abdomen	Other symptoms

SLEEP

How many hours do you sleep on average?	Do you wake up at night & stay awake? How often and how long for?	Do you feel rested when you wake up?
How does it affect your life?	When do you take your last meal of the day?	What makes your sleep better?
What makes your sleep worse?	Women – how does your period affect your sleep?	Do you nap during the day? Does it help you feel better?

STRESS

How would you rate your stress level on a 1-10 scale?	What causes it?	How does it affect your digestion and stool?
How do you cope?	Does it raise or lower your appetite? What foods do you eat when you are stressed?	Does it affect your sleep? How?
Do you smoke/ drink? If yes, do you smoke/drink more when stressed?	Do you meditate, do breathing exercises when stressed?	Do you feel chronically tired?

EXERCISE

Do you exercise? How often and how long for? What type of exercise do you do?	How does it affect your digestion, sleep and overall health?

FOOD INTOLERANCE, ALLERGIES

Do you suffer from food intolerance? What foods are you intolerant to?	Do you suffer from food allergies? What foods are you allergic to?

CURRENT GENERAL HEALTH & PAST ISSUES

Digestive issues	High blood pressure	Heart disease	Diabetes type 2

Diabetes type 1	Epilepsy	Mental health problems	Eating disorders
Self-harm	Operations	Medication taken	Past issues & treatments
Accidents, injuries	Cancer	Pregnancies (women)	Menopause (women)
Fertility issues	High cholesterol	Arthritis, gout	Overweight

CHEMICAL EXPOSURE

Artificial sweeteners	Food additives	Preservatives (processed food & drinks)	Plastics
Tobacco smoke	Car fumes	Medicines	Petroleum products
Cosmetics, beauty products	Pesticides	Paint	Products containing heavy metals
Recreational drugs			

CLIENT'S DIETARY PREFERENCES

Omnivorous	Vegetarian
Vegan	Paleo

Low Carb / Keto	Pescatarian
Frutarian	Other

DIETARY & HEALTH RECOMMENDATIONS

Breakfast	Lunch
Dinner	Snacks
Water	Sleep
Exercise	Relaxation routines
Fasting periods (if any)	Supplements

Note: depending on the client's state of health and food preferences, you may decided to supply the client with a sheet of recommended foods for the week. This, of course, needs to be agreed with the client.

DISCLAIMER

I declare, that all the information regarding me in this form is true and accurate, and as far as I am aware, I can undertake sports massage treatment without adverse effects to my health. I have been fully informed of any contra-indications and I am willing to undertake treatment with this therapist.

Client's signature……………………………...…..Date……………………………………..…..

Therapist's signature…………….............................. Date…………………………………….....

FOLLOW-UP CONSULTATION # 2

Client's name	Address
Therapist's name	Date

STATE OF HEALTH SINCE THE LAST APPOINTMENT

Have the symptoms presented last time improved/ got worse? How have they changed?	
Digestion	
Elimination	
Sleep	
Stress	
Energy levels/ fatigue	
General state of health	
Mental state	

Have you followed the recommendations and agreed diet plan?
_____
_____
_____

What do you think helped you most?
_____
_____
_____

What didn't help?
_____
_____
_____

What changes would you like to make to your diet?
_____
_____
_____

What changes would you like to make to your lifestyle?
_____
_____
_____

AGREED PLAN FOR THE NEXT AGREED PERIOD

Client signature _____ Date_____

FOLLOW-UP CONSULTATION # 3

Client's name	Address
Therapist's name	Date

STATE OF HEALTH SINCE THE LAST APPOINTMENT

Have the symptoms presented last time improved/ got worse? How have they changed?	
Digestion	
Elimination	
Sleep	
Stress	
Energy levels/ fatigue	
General state of health	
Mental state	

Have you followed the recommendations and agreed diet plan?

_____
_____
_____

What do you think helped you most?

_____
_____
_____

What didn't help?

_____
_____
_____

What changes would you like to make to your diet?

_____
_____
_____

What changes would you like to make to your lifestyle?

_____
_____
_____

AGREED PLAN FOR THE NEXT AGREED PERIOD

Client signature _____ Date_____

FOLLOW-UP CONSULTATION # 4

Client's name	Address
Therapist's name	Date

STATE OF HEALTH SINCE THE LAST APPOINTMENT

Have the symptoms presented last time improved/ got worse? How have they changed?	
Digestion	
Elimination	
Sleep	
Stress	
Energy levels/ fatigue	
General state of health	
Mental state	

Have you followed the recommendations and agreed diet plan?
_____
_____
_____

What do you think helped you most?
_____
_____
_____

What didn't help?
_____
_____
_____

What changes would you like to make to your diet?
_____
_____
_____

What changes would you like to make to your lifestyle?
_____
_____
_____

AGREED PLAN FOR THE NEXT AGREED PERIOD

Client signature _____ Date_____

AGREED WEEKLY DIET & HEALTH MANAGEMENT PLAN

Monday

Breakfast	Lunch
Dinner	Snacks
Water	Sleep
Exercise	Relaxation routines
Fasting periods (if any)	Supplements

Tuesday

Breakfast	Lunch
Dinner	Snacks
Water	Sleep
Exercise	Relaxation routines
Fasting periods (if any)	Supplements

Wednesday

Breakfast	Lunch
Dinner	Snacks
Water	Sleep
Exercise	Relaxation routines
Fasting periods (if any)	Supplements

Thursday

Breakfast	Lunch
Dinner	Snacks
Water	Sleep
Exercise	Relaxation routines
Fasting periods (if any)	Supplements

Friday

Breakfast	Lunch
Dinner	Snacks
Water	Sleep
Exercise	Relaxation routines
Fasting periods (if any)	Supplements

Saturday

Breakfast	Lunch
Dinner	Snacks
Water	Sleep
Exercise	Relaxation routines
Fasting periods (if any)	Supplements

Sunday

Breakfast	Lunch
Dinner	Snacks
Water	Sleep
Exercise	Relaxation routines
Fasting periods (if any)	Supplements

Weekly Results & Observations

Therapist's Notes

HOLISTIC NUTRITION CONSULTATION FORM

Therapist:	Clinic:	Date:
Client's name:	Age:	Gender:
Height	Weight	BMI
Client' address: Tel No:	Occupation:	Doctor's address/ telephone no.

CLIENT'S HEALTH OBJECTIVES

WHAT HEALTH ISSUES & SYMPTOMS CONCERN THE CLIENT?

TYPICAL FOODS & DRINKS CONSUMED DURING THE DAY + QUANTITIES

Breakfast	Lunch
Dinner	Snacks between meals
Fruit & vegetables	Water

Other drinks	Supplements (if any)

DIGESTION & ELIMINATION

Slow digestion	Acid reflux	Indigestion	Stomach pain
Bloating	IBS	Wind	Nausea after eating
Stool type & frequency	Undigested food in stool	Pain anywhere else in the abdomen	Other symptoms

SLEEP

How many hours do you sleep on average?	Do you wake up at night & stay awake? How often and how long for?	Do you feel rested when you wake up?
How does it affect your life?	When do you take your last meal of the day?	What makes your sleep better?
What makes your sleep worse?	Women – how does your period affect your sleep?	Do you nap during the day? Does it help you feel better?

STRESS

How would you rate your stress level on a 1-10 scale?	What causes it?	How does it affect your digestion and stool?
How do you cope?	Does it raise or lower your appetite? What foods do you eat when you are stressed?	Does it affect your sleep? How?
Do you smoke/ drink? If yes, do you smoke/drink more when stressed?	Do you meditate, do breathing exercises when stressed?	Do you feel chronically tired?

EXERCISE

Do you exercise? How often and how long for? What type of exercise do you do?	How does it affect your digestion, sleep and overall health?

FOOD INTOLERANCE, ALLERGIES

Do you suffer from food intolerance? What foods are you intolerant to?	Do you suffer from food allergies? What foods are you allergic to?

CURRENT GENERAL HEALTH & PAST ISSUES

Digestive issues	High blood pressure	Heart disease	Diabetes type 2

Diabetes type 1	Epilepsy	Mental health problems	Eating disorders
Self-harm	Operations	Medication taken	Past issues & treatments
Accidents, injuries	Cancer	Pregnancies (women)	Menopause (women)
Fertility issues	High cholesterol	Arthritis, gout	Overweight

CHEMICAL EXPOSURE

Artificial sweeteners	Food additives	Preservatives (processed food & drinks)	Plastics
Tobacco smoke	Car fumes	Medicines	Petroleum products
Cosmetics, beauty products	Pesticides	Paint	Products containing heavy metals
Recreational drugs			

CLIENT'S DIETARY PREFERENCES

Omnivorous	Vegetarian
Vegan	Paleo

Low Carb / Keto	Pescatarian
Frutarian	Other

DIETARY & HEALTH RECOMMENDATIONS

Breakfast	Lunch
Dinner	Snacks
Water	Sleep
Exercise	Relaxation routines
Fasting periods (if any)	Supplements

Note: depending on the client's state of health and food preferences, you may decided to supply the client with a sheet of recommended foods for the week. This, of course, needs to be agreed with the client.

DISCLAIMER

I declare, that all the information regarding me in this form is true and accurate, and as far as I am aware, I can undertake sports massage treatment without adverse effects to my health. I have been fully informed of any contra-indications and I am willing to undertake treatment with this therapist.

Client's signature………………………………..…..Date……………………………………..

Therapist's signature……………..……………………. Date……………………………………..

FOLLOW-UP CONSULTATION # 2

Client's name	Address
Therapist's name	Date

STATE OF HEALTH SINCE THE LAST APPOINTMENT

Have the symptoms presented last time improved/ got worse? How have they changed?	
Digestion	
Elimination	
Sleep	
Stress	
Energy levels/ fatigue	
General state of health	
Mental state	

Have you followed the recommendations and agreed diet plan?
_____
_____
_____

What do you think helped you most?
_____
_____
_____

What didn't help?
_____
_____
_____

What changes would you like to make to your diet?
_____
_____
_____

What changes would you like to make to your lifestyle?
_____
_____
_____

AGREED PLAN FOR THE NEXT AGREED PERIOD

Client signature _____ Date _____

FOLLOW-UP CONSULTATION # 3

Client's name	Address
Therapist's name	Date

STATE OF HEALTH SINCE THE LAST APPOINTMENT

Have the symptoms presented last time improved/ got worse? How have they changed?	
Digestion	
Elimination	
Sleep	
Stress	
Energy levels/ fatigue	
General state of health	
Mental state	

Have you followed the recommendations and agreed diet plan?
_____
_____
_____

What do you think helped you most?
_____
_____
_____

What didn't help?
_____
_____
_____

What changes would you like to make to your diet?
_____
_____
_____

What changes would you like to make to your lifestyle?
_____
_____
_____

AGREED PLAN FOR THE NEXT AGREED PERIOD

Client signature _____ Date_____

FOLLOW-UP CONSULTATION # 4

Client's name	Address
Therapist's name	Date

STATE OF HEALTH SINCE THE LAST APPOINTMENT

Have the symptoms presented last time improved/ got worse? How have they changed?	
Digestion	
Elimination	
Sleep	
Stress	
Energy levels/ fatigue	
General state of health	
Mental state	

Have you followed the recommendations and agreed diet plan?
_____
_____
_____

What do you think helped you most?
_____
_____
_____

What didn't help?
_____
_____
_____

What changes would you like to make to your diet?
_____
_____
_____

What changes would you like to make to your lifestyle?
_____
_____
_____

AGREED PLAN FOR THE NEXT AGREED PERIOD

Client signature _____ Date_____

AGREED WEEKLY DIET & HEALTH MANAGEMENT PLAN

Monday

Breakfast	Lunch
Dinner	Snacks
Water	Sleep
Exercise	Relaxation routines
Fasting periods (if any)	Supplements

Tuesday

Breakfast	Lunch
Dinner	Snacks
Water	Sleep
Exercise	Relaxation routines
Fasting periods (if any)	Supplements

Wednesday

Breakfast	Lunch
Dinner	Snacks
Water	Sleep
Exercise	Relaxation routines
Fasting periods (if any)	Supplements

Thursday

Breakfast	Lunch
Dinner	Snacks
Water	Sleep
Exercise	Relaxation routines
Fasting periods (if any)	Supplements

Friday

Breakfast	Lunch
Dinner	Snacks
Water	Sleep
Exercise	Relaxation routines
Fasting periods (if any)	Supplements

Saturday

Breakfast	Lunch
Dinner	Snacks
Water	Sleep
Exercise	Relaxation routines
Fasting periods (if any)	Supplements

Sunday

Breakfast	Lunch
Dinner	Snacks
Water	Sleep
Exercise	Relaxation routines
Fasting periods (if any)	Supplements

Weekly Results & Observations

Therapist's Notes

HOLISTIC NUTRITION CONSULTATION FORM

Therapist:	Clinic:	Date:
Client's name:	Age:	Gender:
Height	Weight	BMI
Client' address: Tel No:	Occupation:	Doctor's address/ telephone no.

CLIENT'S HEALTH OBJECTIVES

WHAT HEALTH ISSUES & SYMPTOMS CONCERN THE CLIENT?

TYPICAL FOODS & DRINKS CONSUMED DURING THE DAY + QUANTITIES

Breakfast	Lunch
Dinner	Snacks between meals
Fruit & vegetables	Water

Other drinks	Supplements (if any)

DIGESTION & ELIMINATION

Slow digestion	Acid reflux	Indigestion	Stomach pain
Bloating	IBS	Wind	Nausea after eating
Stool type & frequency	Undigested food in stool	Pain anywhere else in the abdomen	Other symptoms

SLEEP

How many hours do you sleep on average?	Do you wake up at night & stay awake? How often and how long for?	Do you feel rested when you wake up?
How does it affect your life?	When do you take your last meal of the day?	What makes your sleep better?
What makes your sleep worse?	Women – how does your period affect your sleep?	Do you nap during the day? Does it help you feel better?

STRESS

How would you rate your stress level on a 1-10 scale?	What causes it?	How does it affect your digestion and stool?
How do you cope?	Does it raise or lower your appetite? What foods do you eat when you are stressed?	Does it affect your sleep? How?
Do you smoke/ drink? If yes, do you smoke/drink more when stressed?	Do you meditate, do breathing exercises when stressed?	Do you feel chronically tired?

EXERCISE

Do you exercise? How often and how long for? What type of exercise do you do?	How does it affect your digestion, sleep and overall health?

FOOD INTOLERANCE, ALLERGIES

Do you suffer from food intolerance? What foods are you intolerant to?	Do you suffer from food allergies? What foods are you allergic to?

CURRENT GENERAL HEALTH & PAST ISSUES

Digestive issues	High blood pressure	Heart disease	Diabetes type 2

Diabetes type 1	Epilepsy	Mental health problems	Eating disorders
Self-harm	Operations	Medication taken	Past issues & treatments
Accidents, injuries	Cancer	Pregnancies (women)	Menopause (women)
Fertility issues	High cholesterol	Arthritis, gout	Overweight

CHEMICAL EXPOSURE

Artificial sweeteners	Food additives	Preservatives (processed food & drinks)	Plastics
Tobacco smoke	Car fumes	Medicines	Petroleum products
Cosmetics, beauty products	Pesticides	Paint	Products containing heavy metals
Recreational drugs			

CLIENT'S DIETARY PREFERENCES

Omnivorous	Vegetarian
Vegan	Paleo

Low Carb / Keto	Pescatarian
Frutarian	Other

DIETARY & HEALTH RECOMMENDATIONS

Breakfast	Lunch
Dinner	Snacks
Water	Sleep
Exercise	Relaxation routines
Fasting periods (if any)	Supplements

Note: depending on the client's state of health and food preferences, you may decided to supply the client with a sheet of recommended foods for the week. This, of course, needs to be agreed with the client.

DISCLAIMER

I declare, that all the information regarding me in this form is true and accurate, and as far as I am aware, I can undertake sports massage treatment without adverse effects to my health. I have been fully informed of any contra-indications and I am willing to undertake treatment with this therapist.

Client's signature..............................…...Date..

Therapist's signature…………................................. Date..

FOLLOW-UP CONSULTATION # 2

Client's name	Address
Therapist's name	Date

STATE OF HEALTH SINCE THE LAST APPOINTMENT

Have the symptoms presented last time improved/ got worse? How have they changed?	
Digestion	
Elimination	
Sleep	
Stress	
Energy levels/ fatigue	
General state of health	
Mental state	

Have you followed the recommendations and agreed diet plan?
_____
_____
_____

What do you think helped you most?
_____
_____
_____

What didn't help?
_____
_____
_____

What changes would you like to make to your diet?
_____
_____
_____

What changes would you like to make to your lifestyle?
_____
_____
_____

AGREED PLAN FOR THE NEXT AGREED PERIOD

Client signature _____ Date_____

FOLLOW-UP CONSULTATION # 3

Client's name	Address
Therapist's name	Date

STATE OF HEALTH SINCE THE LAST APPOINTMENT

Have the symptoms presented last time improved/ got worse? How have they changed?	
Digestion	
Elimination	
Sleep	
Stress	
Energy levels/ fatigue	
General state of health	
Mental state	

Have you followed the recommendations and agreed diet plan?

_____
_____
_____

What do you think helped you most?

_____
_____
_____

What didn't help?

_____
_____
_____

What changes would you like to make to your diet?

_____
_____
_____

What changes would you like to make to your lifestyle?

_____
_____
_____

AGREED PLAN FOR THE NEXT AGREED PERIOD

Client signature _____ Date_____

FOLLOW-UP CONSULTATION # 4

Client's name	Address
Therapist's name	Date

STATE OF HEALTH SINCE THE LAST APPOINTMENT

Have the symptoms presented last time improved/ got worse? How have they changed?	
Digestion	
Elimination	
Sleep	
Stress	
Energy levels/ fatigue	
General state of health	
Mental state	

Have you followed the recommendations and agreed diet plan?
_____
_____
_____

What do you think helped you most?
_____
_____
_____

What didn't help?
_____
_____
_____

What changes would you like to make to your diet?
_____
_____
_____

What changes would you like to make to your lifestyle?
_____
_____
_____

AGREED PLAN FOR THE NEXT AGREED PERIOD

Client signature _____ Date_____

AGREED WEEKLY DIET & HEALTH MANAGEMENT PLAN

Monday

Breakfast	Lunch
Dinner	Snacks
Water	Sleep
Exercise	Relaxation routines
Fasting periods (if any)	Supplements

Tuesday

Breakfast	Lunch
Dinner	Snacks
Water	Sleep
Exercise	Relaxation routines
Fasting periods (if any)	Supplements

Wednesday

Breakfast	Lunch
Dinner	Snacks
Water	Sleep
Exercise	Relaxation routines
Fasting periods (if any)	Supplements

Thursday

Breakfast	Lunch
Dinner	Snacks
Water	Sleep
Exercise	Relaxation routines
Fasting periods (if any)	Supplements

Friday

Breakfast	Lunch
Dinner	Snacks
Water	Sleep
Exercise	Relaxation routines
Fasting periods (if any)	Supplements

Saturday

Breakfast	Lunch
Dinner	Snacks
Water	Sleep
Exercise	Relaxation routines
Fasting periods (if any)	Supplements

Sunday

Breakfast	Lunch
Dinner	Snacks
Water	Sleep
Exercise	Relaxation routines
Fasting periods (if any)	Supplements

Weekly Results & Observations

Therapist's Notes

HOLISTIC NUTRITION CONSULTATION FORM

Therapist:	Clinic:	Date:
Client's name:	Age:	Gender:
Height	Weight	BMI
Client' address: Tel No:	Occupation:	Doctor's address/ telephone no.

CLIENT'S HEALTH OBJECTIVES

WHAT HEALTH ISSUES & SYMPTOMS CONCERN THE CLIENT?

TYPICAL FOODS & DRINKS CONSUMED DURING THE DAY + QUANTITIES

Breakfast	Lunch
Dinner	Snacks between meals
Fruit & vegetables	Water

Other drinks	Supplements (if any)

DIGESTION & ELIMINATION

Slow digestion	Acid reflux	Indigestion	Stomach pain
Bloating	IBS	Wind	Nausea after eating
Stool type & frequency	Undigested food in stool	Pain anywhere else in the abdomen	Other symptoms

SLEEP

How many hours do you sleep on average?	Do you wake up at night & stay awake? How often and how long for?	Do you feel rested when you wake up?
How does it affect your life?	When do you take your last meal of the day?	What makes your sleep better?
What makes your sleep worse?	Women – how does your period affect your sleep?	Do you nap during the day? Does it help you feel better?

STRESS

How would you rate your stress level on a 1-10 scale?	What causes it?	How does it affect your digestion and stool?
How do you cope?	Does it raise or lower your appetite? What foods do you eat when you are stressed?	Does it affect your sleep? How?
Do you smoke/ drink? If yes, do you smoke/drink more when stressed?	Do you meditate, do breathing exercises when stressed?	Do you feel chronically tired?

EXERCISE

Do you exercise? How often and how long for? What type of exercise do you do?	How does it affect your digestion, sleep and overall health?

FOOD INTOLERANCE, ALLERGIES

Do you suffer from food intolerance? What foods are you intolerant to?	Do you suffer from food allergies? What foods are you allergic to?

CURRENT GENERAL HEALTH & PAST ISSUES

Digestive issues	High blood pressure	Heart disease	Diabetes type 2

Diabetes type 1	Epilepsy	Mental health problems	Eating disorders
Self-harm	Operations	Medication taken	Past issues & treatments
Accidents, injuries	Cancer	Pregnancies (women)	Menopause (women)
Fertility issues	High cholesterol	Arthritis, gout	Overweight

CHEMICAL EXPOSURE

Artificial sweeteners	Food additives	Preservatives (processed food & drinks)	Plastics
Tobacco smoke	Car fumes	Medicines	Petroleum products
Cosmetics, beauty products	Pesticides	Paint	Products containing heavy metals
Recreational drugs			

CLIENT'S DIETARY PREFERENCES

Omnivorous	Vegetarian
Vegan	Paleo

Low Carb / Keto	Pescatarian
Frutarian	Other

DIETARY & HEALTH RECOMMENDATIONS

Breakfast	Lunch
Dinner	Snacks
Water	Sleep
Exercise	Relaxation routines
Fasting periods (if any)	Supplements

Note: depending on the client's state of health and food preferences, you may decided to supply the client with a sheet of recommended foods for the week. This, of course, needs to be agreed with the client.

DISCLAIMER

I declare, that all the information regarding me in this form is true and accurate, and as far as I am aware, I can undertake sports massage treatment without adverse effects to my health. I have been fully informed of any contra-indications and I am willing to undertake treatment with this therapist.

Client's signature……………………………..….Date……………………………….…..

Therapist's signature…………….….................... Date…………………………………..

FOLLOW-UP CONSULTATION # 2

Client's name	Address
Therapist's name	Date

STATE OF HEALTH SINCE THE LAST APPOINTMENT

Have the symptoms presented last time improved/ got worse? How have they changed?	
Digestion	
Elimination	
Sleep	
Stress	
Energy levels/ fatigue	
General state of health	
Mental state	

Have you followed the recommendations and agreed diet plan?
_____
_____
_____

What do you think helped you most?
_____
_____
_____

What didn't help?
_____
_____
_____

What changes would you like to make to your diet?
_____
_____
_____

What changes would you like to make to your lifestyle?
_____
_____
_____

AGREED PLAN FOR THE NEXT AGREED PERIOD

Client signature _____ Date_____

FOLLOW-UP CONSULTATION # 3

Client's name	Address
Therapist's name	Date

STATE OF HEALTH SINCE THE LAST APPOINTMENT

Have the symptoms presented last time improved/ got worse? How have they changed?	
Digestion	
Elimination	
Sleep	
Stress	
Energy levels/ fatigue	
General state of health	
Mental state	

Have you followed the recommendations and agreed diet plan?
_____
_____
_____

What do you think helped you most?
_____
_____
_____

What didn't help?
_____
_____
_____

What changes would you like to make to your diet?
_____
_____
_____

What changes would you like to make to your lifestyle?
_____
_____
_____

AGREED PLAN FOR THE NEXT AGREED PERIOD

Client signature _____ Date_____

FOLLOW-UP CONSULTATION # 4

Client's name	Address
Therapist's name	Date

STATE OF HEALTH SINCE THE LAST APPOINTMENT

Have the symptoms presented last time improved/ got worse? How have they changed?	
Digestion	
Elimination	
Sleep	
Stress	
Energy levels/ fatigue	
General state of health	
Mental state	

Have you followed the recommendations and agreed diet plan?
_____
_____
_____

What do you think helped you most?
_____
_____
_____

What didn't help?
_____
_____
_____

What changes would you like to make to your diet?
_____
_____
_____

What changes would you like to make to your lifestyle?
_____
_____
_____

AGREED PLAN FOR THE NEXT AGREED PERIOD

Client signature _____ Date_____

AGREED WEEKLY DIET & HEALTH MANAGEMENT PLAN

Monday

Breakfast	Lunch
Dinner	Snacks
Water	Sleep
Exercise	Relaxation routines
Fasting periods (if any)	Supplements

Tuesday

Breakfast	Lunch
Dinner	Snacks
Water	Sleep
Exercise	Relaxation routines
Fasting periods (if any)	Supplements

Wednesday

Breakfast	Lunch
Dinner	Snacks
Water	Sleep
Exercise	Relaxation routines
Fasting periods (if any)	Supplements

Thursday

Breakfast	Lunch
Dinner	Snacks
Water	Sleep
Exercise	Relaxation routines
Fasting periods (if any)	Supplements

Friday

Breakfast	Lunch
Dinner	Snacks
Water	Sleep
Exercise	Relaxation routines
Fasting periods (if any)	Supplements

Saturday

Breakfast	Lunch
Dinner	Snacks
Water	Sleep
Exercise	Relaxation routines
Fasting periods (if any)	Supplements

Sunday

Breakfast	Lunch
Dinner	Snacks
Water	Sleep
Exercise	Relaxation routines
Fasting periods (if any)	Supplements

Weekly Results & Observations

Therapist's Notes

HOLISTIC NUTRITION CONSULTATION FORM

Therapist:	Clinic:	Date:
Client's name:	Age:	Gender:
Height	Weight	BMI
Client' address: Tel No:	Occupation:	Doctor's address/ telephone no.

CLIENT'S HEALTH OBJECTIVES

WHAT HEALTH ISSUES & SYMPTOMS CONCERN THE CLIENT?

TYPICAL FOODS & DRINKS CONSUMED DURING THE DAY + QUANTITIES

Breakfast	Lunch
Dinner	Snacks between meals
Fruit & vegetables	Water

Other drinks	Supplements (if any)

DIGESTION & ELIMINATION

Slow digestion	Acid reflux	Indigestion	Stomach pain
Bloating	IBS	Wind	Nausea after eating
Stool type & frequency	Undigested food in stool	Pain anywhere else in the abdomen	Other symptoms

SLEEP

How many hours do you sleep on average?	Do you wake up at night & stay awake? How often and how long for?	Do you feel rested when you wake up?
How does it affect your life?	When do you take your last meal of the day?	What makes your sleep better?
What makes your sleep worse?	Women – how does your period affect your sleep?	Do you nap during the day? Does it help you feel better?

STRESS

How would you rate your stress level on a 1-10 scale?	What causes it?	How does it affect your digestion and stool?
How do you cope?	Does it raise or lower your appetite? What foods do you eat when you are stressed?	Does it affect your sleep? How?
Do you smoke/ drink? If yes, do you smoke/drink more when stressed?	Do you meditate, do breathing exercises when stressed?	Do you feel chronically tired?

EXERCISE

Do you exercise? How often and how long for? What type of exercise do you do?	How does it affect your digestion, sleep and overall health?

FOOD INTOLERANCE, ALLERGIES

Do you suffer from food intolerance? What foods are you intolerant to?	Do you suffer from food allergies? What foods are you allergic to?

CURRENT GENERAL HEALTH & PAST ISSUES

Digestive issues	High blood pressure	Heart disease	Diabetes type 2

Diabetes type 1	Epilepsy	Mental health problems	Eating disorders
Self-harm	Operations	Medication taken	Past issues & treatments
Accidents, injuries	Cancer	Pregnancies (women)	Menopause (women)
Fertility issues	High cholesterol	Arthritis, gout	Overweight

CHEMICAL EXPOSURE

Artificial sweeteners	Food additives	Preservatives (processed food & drinks)	Plastics
Tobacco smoke	Car fumes	Medicines	Petroleum products
Cosmetics, beauty products	Pesticides	Paint	Products containing heavy metals
Recreational drugs			

CLIENT'S DIETARY PREFERENCES

Omnivorous	Vegetarian
Vegan	Paleo

Low Carb / Keto	Pescatarian
Frutarian	Other

DIETARY & HEALTH RECOMMENDATIONS

Breakfast	Lunch
Dinner	Snacks
Water	Sleep
Exercise	Relaxation routines
Fasting periods (if any)	Supplements

Note: depending on the client's state of health and food preferences, you may decided to supply the client with a sheet of recommended foods for the week. This, of course, needs to be agreed with the client.

DISCLAIMER

I declare, that all the information regarding me in this form is true and accurate, and as far as I am aware, I can undertake sports massage treatment without adverse effects to my health. I have been fully informed of any contra-indications and I am willing to undertake treatment with this therapist.

Client's signature................................……..Date..

Therapist's signature…………….............................. Date....................................

FOLLOW-UP CONSULTATION # 2

Client's name	Address
Therapist's name	Date

STATE OF HEALTH SINCE THE LAST APPOINTMENT

Have the symptoms presented last time improved/ got worse? How have they changed?	
Digestion	
Elimination	
Sleep	
Stress	
Energy levels/ fatigue	
General state of health	
Mental state	

Have you followed the recommendations and agreed diet plan?

_____
_____
_____

What do you think helped you most?

_____
_____
_____

What didn't help?

_____
_____
_____

What changes would you like to make to your diet?

_____
_____
_____

What changes would you like to make to your lifestyle?

_____
_____
_____

AGREED PLAN FOR THE NEXT AGREED PERIOD

Client signature _____ Date_____

FOLLOW-UP CONSULTATION # 3

Client's name	Address
Therapist's name	Date

STATE OF HEALTH SINCE THE LAST APPOINTMENT

Have the symptoms presented last time improved/ got worse? How have they changed?	
Digestion	
Elimination	
Sleep	
Stress	
Energy levels/ fatigue	
General state of health	
Mental state	

Have you followed the recommendations and agreed diet plan?
_____
_____
_____

What do you think helped you most?
_____
_____
_____

What didn't help?
_____
_____
_____

What changes would you like to make to your diet?
_____
_____
_____

What changes would you like to make to your lifestyle?
_____
_____
_____

AGREED PLAN FOR THE NEXT AGREED PERIOD

Client signature _____ Date_____

FOLLOW-UP CONSULTATION # 4

Client's name	Address
Therapist's name	Date

STATE OF HEALTH SINCE THE LAST APPOINTMENT

Have the symptoms presented last time improved/ got worse? How have they changed?	
Digestion	
Elimination	
Sleep	
Stress	
Energy levels/ fatigue	
General state of health	
Mental state	

Have you followed the recommendations and agreed diet plan?
_____
_____
_____

What do you think helped you most?
_____
_____
_____

What didn't help?
_____
_____
_____

What changes would you like to make to your diet?
_____
_____
_____

What changes would you like to make to your lifestyle?
_____
_____
_____

AGREED PLAN FOR THE NEXT AGREED PERIOD

Client signature _____ Date_____

AGREED WEEKLY DIET & HEALTH MANAGEMENT PLAN

Monday

Breakfast	Lunch
Dinner	Snacks
Water	Sleep
Exercise	Relaxation routines
Fasting periods (if any)	Supplements

Tuesday

Breakfast	Lunch
Dinner	Snacks
Water	Sleep
Exercise	Relaxation routines
Fasting periods (if any)	Supplements

Wednesday

Breakfast	Lunch
Dinner	Snacks
Water	Sleep
Exercise	Relaxation routines
Fasting periods (if any)	Supplements

Thursday

Breakfast	Lunch
Dinner	Snacks
Water	Sleep
Exercise	Relaxation routines
Fasting periods (if any)	Supplements

Friday

Breakfast	Lunch
Dinner	Snacks
Water	Sleep
Exercise	Relaxation routines
Fasting periods (if any)	Supplements

Saturday

Breakfast	Lunch
Dinner	Snacks
Water	Sleep
Exercise	Relaxation routines
Fasting periods (if any)	Supplements

Sunday

Breakfast	Lunch
Dinner	Snacks
Water	Sleep
Exercise	Relaxation routines
Fasting periods (if any)	Supplements

Weekly Results & Observations

Therapist's Notes

HOLISTIC NUTRITION CONSULTATION FORM

Therapist:	Clinic:	Date:
Client's name:	Age:	Gender:
Height	Weight	BMI
Client' address: Tel No:	Occupation:	Doctor's address/ telephone no.

CLIENT'S HEALTH OBJECTIVES

WHAT HEALTH ISSUES & SYMPTOMS CONCERN THE CLIENT?

TYPICAL FOODS & DRINKS CONSUMED DURING THE DAY + QUANTITIES

Breakfast	Lunch
Dinner	Snacks between meals
Fruit & vegetables	Water

Other drinks	Supplements (if any)

DIGESTION & ELIMINATION

Slow digestion	Acid reflux	Indigestion	Stomach pain
Bloating	IBS	Wind	Nausea after eating
Stool type & frequency	Undigested food in stool	Pain anywhere else in the abdomen	Other symptoms

SLEEP

How many hours do you sleep on average?	Do you wake up at night & stay awake? How often and how long for?	Do you feel rested when you wake up?
How does it affect your life?	When do you take your last meal of the day?	What makes your sleep better?
What makes your sleep worse?	Women – how does your period affect your sleep?	Do you nap during the day? Does it help you feel better?

STRESS

How would you rate your stress level on a 1-10 scale?	What causes it?	How does it affect your digestion and stool?
How do you cope?	Does it raise or lower your appetite? What foods do you eat when you are stressed?	Does it affect your sleep? How?
Do you smoke/ drink? If yes, do you smoke/drink more when stressed?	Do you meditate, do breathing exercises when stressed?	Do you feel chronically tired?

EXERCISE

Do you exercise? How often and how long for? What type of exercise do you do?	How does it affect your digestion, sleep and overall health?

FOOD INTOLERANCE, ALLERGIES

Do you suffer from food intolerance? What foods are you intolerant to?	Do you suffer from food allergies? What foods are you allergic to?

CURRENT GENERAL HEALTH & PAST ISSUES

Digestive issues	High blood pressure	Heart disease	Diabetes type 2

Diabetes type 1	Epilepsy	Mental health problems	Eating disorders
Self-harm	Operations	Medication taken	Past issues & treatments
Accidents, injuries	Cancer	Pregnancies (women)	Menopause (women)
Fertility issues	High cholesterol	Arthritis, gout	Overweight

CHEMICAL EXPOSURE

Artificial sweeteners	Food additives	Preservatives (processed food & drinks)	Plastics
Tobacco smoke	Car fumes	Medicines	Petroleum products
Cosmetics, beauty products	Pesticides	Paint	Products containing heavy metals
Recreational drugs			

CLIENT'S DIETARY PREFERENCES

Omnivorous	Vegetarian
Vegan	Paleo

Low Carb / Keto	Pescatarian
Frutarian	Other

DIETARY & HEALTH RECOMMENDATIONS

Breakfast	Lunch
Dinner	Snacks
Water	Sleep
Exercise	Relaxation routines
Fasting periods (if any)	Supplements

Note: depending on the client's state of health and food preferences, you may decided to supply the client with a sheet of recommended foods for the week. This, of course, needs to be agreed with the client.

DISCLAIMER

I declare, that all the information regarding me in this form is true and accurate, and as far as I am aware, I can undertake sports massage treatment without adverse effects to my health. I have been fully informed of any contra-indications and I am willing to undertake treatment with this therapist.

Client's signature..............................……...Date...…..

Therapist's signature………………................... Date...

FOLLOW-UP CONSULTATION # 2

Client's name	Address
Therapist's name	Date

STATE OF HEALTH SINCE THE LAST APPOINTMENT

Have the symptoms presented last time improved/ got worse? How have they changed?	
Digestion	
Elimination	
Sleep	
Stress	
Energy levels/ fatigue	
General state of health	
Mental state	

Have you followed the recommendations and agreed diet plan?
_____
_____
_____

What do you think helped you most?
_____
_____
_____

What didn't help?
_____
_____
_____

What changes would you like to make to your diet?
_____
_____
_____

What changes would you like to make to your lifestyle?
_____
_____
_____

AGREED PLAN FOR THE NEXT AGREED PERIOD

Client signature _____ Date_____

FOLLOW-UP CONSULTATION # 3

Client's name	Address
Therapist's name	Date

STATE OF HEALTH SINCE THE LAST APPOINTMENT

Have the symptoms presented last time improved/ got worse? How have they changed?	
Digestion	
Elimination	
Sleep	
Stress	
Energy levels/ fatigue	
General state of health	
Mental state	

Have you followed the recommendations and agreed diet plan?

_____
_____
_____

What do you think helped you most?

_____
_____
_____

What didn't help?

_____
_____
_____

What changes would you like to make to your diet?

_____
_____
_____

What changes would you like to make to your lifestyle?

_____
_____
_____

AGREED PLAN FOR THE NEXT AGREED PERIOD

Client signature _____ Date_____

FOLLOW-UP CONSULTATION # 4

Client's name	Address
Therapist's name	Date

STATE OF HEALTH SINCE THE LAST APPOINTMENT

Have the symptoms presented last time improved/ got worse? How have they changed?	
Digestion	
Elimination	
Sleep	
Stress	
Energy levels/ fatigue	
General state of health	
Mental state	

Have you followed the recommendations and agreed diet plan?
_____
_____
_____

What do you think helped you most?
_____
_____
_____

What didn't help?
_____
_____
_____

What changes would you like to make to your diet?
_____
_____
_____

What changes would you like to make to your lifestyle?
_____
_____
_____

AGREED PLAN FOR THE NEXT AGREED PERIOD

+---+
| |
| |
| |
| |
+---+

Client signature _____ Date_____

AGREED WEEKLY DIET & HEALTH MANAGEMENT PLAN

Monday

Breakfast	Lunch
Dinner	Snacks
Water	Sleep
Exercise	Relaxation routines
Fasting periods (if any)	Supplements

Tuesday

Breakfast	Lunch
Dinner	Snacks
Water	Sleep
Exercise	Relaxation routines
Fasting periods (if any)	Supplements

Wednesday

Breakfast	Lunch
Dinner	Snacks
Water	Sleep
Exercise	Relaxation routines
Fasting periods (if any)	Supplements

Thursday

Breakfast	Lunch
Dinner	Snacks
Water	Sleep
Exercise	Relaxation routines
Fasting periods (if any)	Supplements

Friday

Breakfast	Lunch
Dinner	Snacks
Water	Sleep
Exercise	Relaxation routines
Fasting periods (if any)	Supplements

Saturday

Breakfast	Lunch
Dinner	Snacks
Water	Sleep
Exercise	Relaxation routines
Fasting periods (if any)	Supplements

Sunday

Breakfast	Lunch
Dinner	Snacks
Water	Sleep
Exercise	Relaxation routines
Fasting periods (if any)	Supplements

Weekly Results & Observations

Therapist's Notes

HOLISTIC NUTRITION CONSULTATION FORM

Therapist:	Clinic:	Date:
Client's name:	Age:	Gender:
Height	Weight	BMI
Client' address: Tel No:	Occupation:	Doctor's address/ telephone no.

CLIENT'S HEALTH OBJECTIVES

WHAT HEALTH ISSUES & SYMPTOMS CONCERN THE CLIENT?

TYPICAL FOODS & DRINKS CONSUMED DURING THE DAY + QUANTITIES

Breakfast	Lunch
Dinner	Snacks between meals
Fruit & vegetables	Water

Other drinks	Supplements (if any)

DIGESTION & ELIMINATION

Slow digestion	Acid reflux	Indigestion	Stomach pain
Bloating	IBS	Wind	Nausea after eating
Stool type & frequency	Undigested food in stool	Pain anywhere else in the abdomen	Other symptoms

SLEEP

How many hours do you sleep on average?	Do you wake up at night & stay awake? How often and how long for?	Do you feel rested when you wake up?
How does it affect your life?	When do you take your last meal of the day?	What makes your sleep better?
What makes your sleep worse?	Women – how does your period affect your sleep?	Do you nap during the day? Does it help you feel better?

STRESS

How would you rate your stress level on a 1-10 scale?	What causes it?	How does it affect your digestion and stool?
How do you cope?	Does it raise or lower your appetite? What foods do you eat when you are stressed?	Does it affect your sleep? How?
Do you smoke/ drink? If yes, do you smoke/drink more when stressed?	Do you meditate, do breathing exercises when stressed?	Do you feel chronically tired?

EXERCISE

Do you exercise? How often and how long for? What type of exercise do you do?	How does it affect your digestion, sleep and overall health?

FOOD INTOLERANCE, ALLERGIES

Do you suffer from food intolerance? What foods are you intolerant to?	Do you suffer from food allergies? What foods are you allergic to?

CURRENT GENERAL HEALTH & PAST ISSUES

Digestive issues	High blood pressure	Heart disease	Diabetes type 2

Diabetes type 1	Epilepsy	Mental health problems	Eating disorders
Self-harm	Operations	Medication taken	Past issues & treatments
Accidents, injuries	Cancer	Pregnancies (women)	Menopause (women)
Fertility issues	High cholesterol	Arthritis, gout	Overweight

CHEMICAL EXPOSURE

Artificial sweeteners	Food additives	Preservatives (processed food & drinks)	Plastics
Tobacco smoke	Car fumes	Medicines	Petroleum products
Cosmetics, beauty products	Pesticides	Paint	Products containing heavy metals
Recreational drugs			

CLIENT'S DIETARY PREFERENCES

Omnivorous	Vegetarian
Vegan	Paleo

Low Carb / Keto	Pescatarian
Frutarian	Other

DIETARY & HEALTH RECOMMENDATIONS

Breakfast	Lunch
Dinner	Snacks
Water	Sleep
Exercise	Relaxation routines
Fasting periods (if any)	Supplements

Note: depending on the client's state of health and food preferences, you may decided to supply the client with a sheet of recommended foods for the week. This, of course, needs to be agreed with the client.

DISCLAIMER

I declare, that all the information regarding me in this form is true and accurate, and as far as I am aware, I can undertake sports massage treatment without adverse effects to my health. I have been fully informed of any contra-indications and I am willing to undertake treatment with this therapist.

Client's signature..................................……...Date..….

Therapist's signature………….................................. Date..

FOLLOW-UP CONSULTATION # 2

Client's name	Address
Therapist's name	Date

STATE OF HEALTH SINCE THE LAST APPOINTMENT

Have the symptoms presented last time improved/ got worse? How have they changed?	
Digestion	
Elimination	
Sleep	
Stress	
Energy levels/ fatigue	
General state of health	
Mental state	

Have you followed the recommendations and agreed diet plan?
_____
_____
_____

What do you think helped you most?
_____
_____
_____

What didn't help?
_____
_____
_____

What changes would you like to make to your diet?
_____
_____
_____

What changes would you like to make to your lifestyle?
_____
_____
_____

AGREED PLAN FOR THE NEXT AGREED PERIOD

Client signature _____ Date_____

FOLLOW-UP CONSULTATION # 3

Client's name	Address
Therapist's name	Date

STATE OF HEALTH SINCE THE LAST APPOINTMENT

Have the symptoms presented last time improved/ got worse? How have they changed?	
Digestion	
Elimination	
Sleep	
Stress	
Energy levels/ fatigue	
General state of health	
Mental state	

Have you followed the recommendations and agreed diet plan?
_____
_____
_____

What do you think helped you most?
_____
_____
_____

What didn't help?
_____
_____
_____

What changes would you like to make to your diet?
_____
_____
_____

What changes would you like to make to your lifestyle?
_____
_____
_____

AGREED PLAN FOR THE NEXT AGREED PERIOD

Client signature _____ Date_____

FOLLOW-UP CONSULTATION # 4

Client's name	Address
Therapist's name	Date

STATE OF HEALTH SINCE THE LAST APPOINTMENT

Have the symptoms presented last time improved/ got worse? How have they changed?	
Digestion	
Elimination	
Sleep	
Stress	
Energy levels/ fatigue	
General state of health	
Mental state	

Have you followed the recommendations and agreed diet plan?
_____
_____
_____

What do you think helped you most?
_____
_____
_____

What didn't help?
_____
_____
_____

What changes would you like to make to your diet?
_____
_____
_____

What changes would you like to make to your lifestyle?
_____
_____
_____

AGREED PLAN FOR THE NEXT AGREED PERIOD

Client signature _____ Date_____

AGREED WEEKLY DIET & HEALTH MANAGEMENT PLAN

Monday

Breakfast	Lunch
Dinner	Snacks
Water	Sleep
Exercise	Relaxation routines
Fasting periods (if any)	Supplements

Tuesday

Breakfast	Lunch
Dinner	Snacks
Water	Sleep
Exercise	Relaxation routines
Fasting periods (if any)	Supplements

Wednesday

Breakfast	Lunch
Dinner	Snacks
Water	Sleep
Exercise	Relaxation routines
Fasting periods (if any)	Supplements

Thursday

Breakfast	Lunch
Dinner	Snacks
Water	Sleep
Exercise	Relaxation routines
Fasting periods (if any)	Supplements

Friday

Breakfast	Lunch
Dinner	Snacks
Water	Sleep
Exercise	Relaxation routines
Fasting periods (if any)	Supplements

Saturday

Breakfast	Lunch
Dinner	Snacks
Water	Sleep
Exercise	Relaxation routines
Fasting periods (if any)	Supplements

Sunday

Breakfast	Lunch
Dinner	Snacks
Water	Sleep
Exercise	Relaxation routines
Fasting periods (if any)	Supplements

Weekly Results & Observations

Therapist's Notes

HOLISTIC NUTRITION CONSULTATION FORM

Therapist:	Clinic:	Date:
Client's name:	Age:	Gender:
Height	Weight	BMI
Client' address: Tel No:	Occupation:	Doctor's address/ telephone no.

CLIENT'S HEALTH OBJECTIVES

WHAT HEALTH ISSUES & SYMPTOMS CONCERN THE CLIENT?

TYPICAL FOODS & DRINKS CONSUMED DURING THE DAY + QUANTITIES

Breakfast	Lunch
Dinner	Snacks between meals
Fruit & vegetables	Water

Other drinks	Supplements (if any)

DIGESTION & ELIMINATION

Slow digestion	Acid reflux	Indigestion	Stomach pain
Bloating	IBS	Wind	Nausea after eating
Stool type & frequency	Undigested food in stool	Pain anywhere else in the abdomen	Other symptoms

SLEEP

How many hours do you sleep on average?	Do you wake up at night & stay awake? How often and how long for?	Do you feel rested when you wake up?
How does it affect your life?	When do you take your last meal of the day?	What makes your sleep better?
What makes your sleep worse?	Women – how does your period affect your sleep?	Do you nap during the day? Does it help you feel better?

STRESS

How would you rate your stress level on a 1-10 scale?	What causes it?	How does it affect your digestion and stool?
How do you cope?	Does it raise or lower your appetite? What foods do you eat when you are stressed?	Does it affect your sleep? How?
Do you smoke/ drink? If yes, do you smoke/drink more when stressed?	Do you meditate, do breathing exercises when stressed?	Do you feel chronically tired?

EXERCISE

Do you exercise? How often and how long for? What type of exercise do you do?	How does it affect your digestion, sleep and overall health?

FOOD INTOLERANCE, ALLERGIES

Do you suffer from food intolerance? What foods are you intolerant to?	Do you suffer from food allergies? What foods are you allergic to?

CURRENT GENERAL HEALTH & PAST ISSUES

Digestive issues	High blood pressure	Heart disease	Diabetes type 2

Diabetes type 1	Epilepsy	Mental health problems	Eating disorders
Self-harm	Operations	Medication taken	Past issues & treatments
Accidents, injuries	Cancer	Pregnancies (women)	Menopause (women)
Fertility issues	High cholesterol	Arthritis, gout	Overweight

CHEMICAL EXPOSURE

Artificial sweeteners	Food additives	Preservatives (processed food & drinks)	Plastics
Tobacco smoke	Car fumes	Medicines	Petroleum products
Cosmetics, beauty products	Pesticides	Paint	Products containing heavy metals
Recreational drugs			

CLIENT'S DIETARY PREFERENCES

Omnivorous	Vegetarian
Vegan	Paleo

Low Carb / Keto	Pescatarian
Frutarian	Other

DIETARY & HEALTH RECOMMENDATIONS

Breakfast	Lunch
Dinner	Snacks
Water	Sleep
Exercise	Relaxation routines
Fasting periods (if any)	Supplements

Note: depending on the client's state of health and food preferences, you may decided to supply the client with a sheet of recommended foods for the week. This, of course, needs to be agreed with the client.

DISCLAIMER

I declare, that all the information regarding me in this form is true and accurate, and as far as I am aware, I can undertake sports massage treatment without adverse effects to my health. I have been fully informed of any contra-indications and I am willing to undertake treatment with this therapist.

Client's signature………………………………...…..Date……………………………………...….

Therapist's signature…………….............................. Date……………………………………...

FOLLOW-UP CONSULTATION # 2

Client's name	Address
Therapist's name	Date

STATE OF HEALTH SINCE THE LAST APPOINTMENT

Have the symptoms presented last time improved/ got worse? How have they changed?	
Digestion	
Elimination	
Sleep	
Stress	
Energy levels/ fatigue	
General state of health	
Mental state	

Have you followed the recommendations and agreed diet plan?
_____
_____
_____

What do you think helped you most?
_____
_____
_____

What didn't help?
_____
_____
_____

What changes would you like to make to your diet?
_____
_____
_____

What changes would you like to make to your lifestyle?
_____
_____
_____

AGREED PLAN FOR THE NEXT AGREED PERIOD

Client signature _____ Date_____

FOLLOW-UP CONSULTATION # 3

Client's name	Address
Therapist's name	Date

STATE OF HEALTH SINCE THE LAST APPOINTMENT

Have the symptoms presented last time improved/ got worse? How have they changed?	
Digestion	
Elimination	
Sleep	
Stress	
Energy levels/ fatigue	
General state of health	
Mental state	

Have you followed the recommendations and agreed diet plan?
_____
_____
_____

What do you think helped you most?
_____
_____
_____

What didn't help?
_____
_____
_____

What changes would you like to make to your diet?
_____
_____
_____

What changes would you like to make to your lifestyle?
_____
_____
_____

AGREED PLAN FOR THE NEXT AGREED PERIOD

Client signature _____ Date_____

FOLLOW-UP CONSULTATION # 4

Client's name	Address
Therapist's name	Date

STATE OF HEALTH SINCE THE LAST APPOINTMENT

Have the symptoms presented last time improved/ got worse? How have they changed?	
Digestion	
Elimination	
Sleep	
Stress	
Energy levels/ fatigue	
General state of health	
Mental state	

Have you followed the recommendations and agreed diet plan?
_____
_____
_____

What do you think helped you most?
_____
_____
_____

What didn't help?
_____
_____
_____

What changes would you like to make to your diet?
_____
_____
_____

What changes would you like to make to your lifestyle?
_____
_____
_____

AGREED PLAN FOR THE NEXT AGREED PERIOD

Client signature _____ Date_____

AGREED WEEKLY DIET & HEALTH MANAGEMENT PLAN

Monday

Breakfast	Lunch
Dinner	Snacks
Water	Sleep
Exercise	Relaxation routines
Fasting periods (if any)	Supplements

Tuesday

Breakfast	Lunch
Dinner	Snacks
Water	Sleep
Exercise	Relaxation routines
Fasting periods (if any)	Supplements

Wednesday

Breakfast	Lunch
Dinner	Snacks
Water	Sleep
Exercise	Relaxation routines
Fasting periods (if any)	Supplements

Thursday

Breakfast	Lunch
Dinner	Snacks
Water	Sleep
Exercise	Relaxation routines
Fasting periods (if any)	Supplements

Friday

Breakfast	Lunch
Dinner	Snacks
Water	Sleep
Exercise	Relaxation routines
Fasting periods (if any)	Supplements

Saturday

Breakfast	Lunch
Dinner	Snacks
Water	Sleep
Exercise	Relaxation routines
Fasting periods (if any)	Supplements

Sunday

Breakfast	Lunch
Dinner	Snacks
Water	Sleep
Exercise	Relaxation routines
Fasting periods (if any)	Supplements

Weekly Results & Observations

Therapist's Notes

HOLISTIC NUTRITION CONSULTATION FORM

Therapist:	Clinic:	Date:
Client's name:	Age:	Gender:
Height	Weight	BMI
Client' address: Tel No:	Occupation:	Doctor's address/ telephone no.

CLIENT'S HEALTH OBJECTIVES

WHAT HEALTH ISSUES & SYMPTOMS CONCERN THE CLIENT?

TYPICAL FOODS & DRINKS CONSUMED DURING THE DAY + QUANTITIES

Breakfast	Lunch
Dinner	Snacks between meals
Fruit & vegetables	Water

Other drinks	Supplements (if any)

DIGESTION & ELIMINATION

Slow digestion	Acid reflux	Indigestion	Stomach pain
Bloating	IBS	Wind	Nausea after eating
Stool type & frequency	Undigested food in stool	Pain anywhere else in the abdomen	Other symptoms

SLEEP

How many hours do you sleep on average?	Do you wake up at night & stay awake? How often and how long for?	Do you feel rested when you wake up?
How does it affect your life?	When do you take your last meal of the day?	What makes your sleep better?
What makes your sleep worse?	Women – how does your period affect your sleep?	Do you nap during the day? Does it help you feel better?

STRESS

How would you rate your stress level on a 1-10 scale?	What causes it?	How does it affect your digestion and stool?
How do you cope?	Does it raise or lower your appetite? What foods do you eat when you are stressed?	Does it affect your sleep? How?
Do you smoke/ drink? If yes, do you smoke/drink more when stressed?	Do you meditate, do breathing exercises when stressed?	Do you feel chronically tired?

EXERCISE

Do you exercise? How often and how long for? What type of exercise do you do?	How does it affect your digestion, sleep and overall health?

FOOD INTOLERANCE, ALLERGIES

Do you suffer from food intolerance? What foods are you intolerant to?	Do you suffer from food allergies? What foods are you allergic to?

CURRENT GENERAL HEALTH & PAST ISSUES

Digestive issues	High blood pressure	Heart disease	Diabetes type 2

Diabetes type 1	Epilepsy	Mental health problems	Eating disorders
Self-harm	Operations	Medication taken	Past issues & treatments
Accidents, injuries	Cancer	Pregnancies (women)	Menopause (women)
Fertility issues	High cholesterol	Arthritis, gout	Overweight

CHEMICAL EXPOSURE

Artificial sweeteners	Food additives	Preservatives (processed food & drinks)	Plastics
Tobacco smoke	Car fumes	Medicines	Petroleum products
Cosmetics, beauty products	Pesticides	Paint	Products containing heavy metals
Recreational drugs			

CLIENT'S DIETARY PREFERENCES

Omnivorous	Vegetarian
Vegan	Paleo

Low Carb / Keto	Pescatarian
Frutarian	Other

DIETARY & HEALTH RECOMMENDATIONS

Breakfast	Lunch
Dinner	Snacks
Water	Sleep
Exercise	Relaxation routines
Fasting periods (if any)	Supplements

Note: depending on the client's state of health and food preferences, you may decided to supply the client with a sheet of recommended foods for the week. This, of course, needs to be agreed with the client.

DISCLAIMER

I declare, that all the information regarding me in this form is true and accurate, and as far as I am aware, I can undertake sports massage treatment without adverse effects to my health. I have been fully informed of any contra-indications and I am willing to undertake treatment with this therapist.

Client's signature...Date..

Therapist's signature.. Date..

FOLLOW-UP CONSULTATION # 2

Client's name	Address
Therapist's name	Date

STATE OF HEALTH SINCE THE LAST APPOINTMENT

Have the symptoms presented last time improved/ got worse? How have they changed?	
Digestion	
Elimination	
Sleep	
Stress	
Energy levels/ fatigue	
General state of health	
Mental state	

Have you followed the recommendations and agreed diet plan?
_____
_____
_____

What do you think helped you most?
_____
_____
_____

What didn't help?
_____
_____
_____

What changes would you like to make to your diet?
_____
_____
_____

What changes would you like to make to your lifestyle?
_____
_____
_____

AGREED PLAN FOR THE NEXT AGREED PERIOD

Client signature _____ Date_____

FOLLOW-UP CONSULTATION # 3

Client's name	Address
Therapist's name	Date

STATE OF HEALTH SINCE THE LAST APPOINTMENT

Have the symptoms presented last time improved/ got worse? How have they changed?	
Digestion	
Elimination	
Sleep	
Stress	
Energy levels/ fatigue	
General state of health	
Mental state	

Have you followed the recommendations and agreed diet plan?
_____
_____
_____

What do you think helped you most?
_____
_____
_____

What didn't help?
_____
_____
_____

What changes would you like to make to your diet?
_____
_____
_____

What changes would you like to make to your lifestyle?
_____
_____
_____

AGREED PLAN FOR THE NEXT AGREED PERIOD

Client signature _____ Date_____

FOLLOW-UP CONSULTATION # 4

Client's name	Address
Therapist's name	Date

STATE OF HEALTH SINCE THE LAST APPOINTMENT

Have the symptoms presented last time improved/ got worse? How have they changed?	
Digestion	
Elimination	
Sleep	
Stress	
Energy levels/ fatigue	
General state of health	
Mental state	

Have you followed the recommendations and agreed diet plan?
_____
_____
_____

What do you think helped you most?
_____
_____
_____

What didn't help?
_____
_____
_____

What changes would you like to make to your diet?
_____
_____
_____

What changes would you like to make to your lifestyle?
_____
_____
_____

AGREED PLAN FOR THE NEXT AGREED PERIOD

Client signature _____ Date_____

AGREED WEEKLY DIET & HEALTH MANAGEMENT PLAN

Monday

Breakfast	Lunch
Dinner	Snacks
Water	Sleep
Exercise	Relaxation routines
Fasting periods (if any)	Supplements

Tuesday

Breakfast	Lunch
Dinner	Snacks
Water	Sleep
Exercise	Relaxation routines
Fasting periods (if any)	Supplements

Wednesday

Breakfast	Lunch
Dinner	Snacks
Water	Sleep
Exercise	Relaxation routines
Fasting periods (if any)	Supplements

Thursday

Breakfast	Lunch
Dinner	Snacks
Water	Sleep
Exercise	Relaxation routines
Fasting periods (if any)	Supplements

Friday

Breakfast	Lunch
Dinner	Snacks
Water	Sleep
Exercise	Relaxation routines
Fasting periods (if any)	Supplements

Saturday

Breakfast	Lunch
Dinner	Snacks
Water	Sleep
Exercise	Relaxation routines
Fasting periods (if any)	Supplements

Sunday

Breakfast	Lunch
Dinner	Snacks
Water	Sleep
Exercise	Relaxation routines
Fasting periods (if any)	Supplements

Weekly Results & Observations

Therapist's Notes

HOLISTIC NUTRITION CONSULTATION FORM

Therapist:	Clinic:	Date:
Client's name:	Age:	Gender:
Height	Weight	BMI
Client' address: Tel No:	Occupation:	Doctor's address/ telephone no.

CLIENT'S HEALTH OBJECTIVES

WHAT HEALTH ISSUES & SYMPTOMS CONCERN THE CLIENT?

TYPICAL FOODS & DRINKS CONSUMED DURING THE DAY + QUANTITIES

Breakfast	Lunch
Dinner	Snacks between meals
Fruit & vegetables	Water

Other drinks	Supplements (if any)

DIGESTION & ELIMINATION

Slow digestion	Acid reflux	Indigestion	Stomach pain
Bloating	IBS	Wind	Nausea after eating
Stool type & frequency	Undigested food in stool	Pain anywhere else in the abdomen	Other symptoms

SLEEP

How many hours do you sleep on average?	Do you wake up at night & stay awake? How often and how long for?	Do you feel rested when you wake up?
How does it affect your life?	When do you take your last meal of the day?	What makes your sleep better?
What makes your sleep worse?	Women – how does your period affect your sleep?	Do you nap during the day? Does it help you feel better?

STRESS

How would you rate your stress level on a 1-10 scale?	What causes it?	How does it affect your digestion and stool?
How do you cope?	Does it raise or lower your appetite? What foods do you eat when you are stressed?	Does it affect your sleep? How?
Do you smoke/ drink? If yes, do you smoke/drink more when stressed?	Do you meditate, do breathing exercises when stressed?	Do you feel chronically tired?

EXERCISE

Do you exercise? How often and how long for? What type of exercise do you do?	How does it affect your digestion, sleep and overall health?

FOOD INTOLERANCE, ALLERGIES

Do you suffer from food intolerance? What foods are you intolerant to?	Do you suffer from food allergies? What foods are you allergic to?

CURRENT GENERAL HEALTH & PAST ISSUES

Digestive issues	High blood pressure	Heart disease	Diabetes type 2

Diabetes type 1	Epilepsy	Mental health problems	Eating disorders
Self-harm	Operations	Medication taken	Past issues & treatments
Accidents, injuries	Cancer	Pregnancies (women)	Menopause (women)
Fertility issues	High cholesterol	Arthritis, gout	Overweight

CHEMICAL EXPOSURE

Artificial sweeteners	Food additives	Preservatives (processed food & drinks)	Plastics
Tobacco smoke	Car fumes	Medicines	Petroleum products
Cosmetics, beauty products	Pesticides	Paint	Products containing heavy metals
Recreational drugs			

CLIENT'S DIETARY PREFERENCES

Omnivorous	Vegetarian
Vegan	Paleo

Low Carb / Keto	Pescatarian
Frutarian	Other

DIETARY & HEALTH RECOMMENDATIONS

Breakfast	Lunch
Dinner	Snacks
Water	Sleep
Exercise	Relaxation routines
Fasting periods (if any)	Supplements

Note: depending on the client's state of health and food preferences, you may decided to supply the client with a sheet of recommended foods for the week. This, of course, needs to be agreed with the client.

DISCLAIMER

I declare, that all the information regarding me in this form is true and accurate, and as far as I am aware, I can undertake sports massage treatment without adverse effects to my health. I have been fully informed of any contra-indications and I am willing to undertake treatment with this therapist.

Client's signature………………………………..Date……………………………………..

Therapist's signature………………............................ Date..

FOLLOW-UP CONSULTATION # 2

Client's name	Address
Therapist's name	Date

STATE OF HEALTH SINCE THE LAST APPOINTMENT

Have the symptoms presented last time improved/ got worse? How have they changed?	
Digestion	
Elimination	
Sleep	
Stress	
Energy levels/ fatigue	
General state of health	
Mental state	

Have you followed the recommendations and agreed diet plan?
_____
_____
_____

What do you think helped you most?
_____
_____
_____

What didn't help?
_____
_____
_____

What changes would you like to make to your diet?
_____
_____
_____

What changes would you like to make to your lifestyle?
_____
_____
_____

AGREED PLAN FOR THE NEXT AGREED PERIOD

Client signature _____ Date_____

FOLLOW-UP CONSULTATION # 3

Client's name	Address
Therapist's name	Date

STATE OF HEALTH SINCE THE LAST APPOINTMENT

Have the symptoms presented last time improved/ got worse? How have they changed?	
Digestion	
Elimination	
Sleep	
Stress	
Energy levels/ fatigue	
General state of health	
Mental state	

Have you followed the recommendations and agreed diet plan?
_____
_____
_____

What do you think helped you most?
_____
_____
_____

What didn't help?
_____
_____
_____

What changes would you like to make to your diet?
_____
_____
_____

What changes would you like to make to your lifestyle?
_____
_____
_____

AGREED PLAN FOR THE NEXT AGREED PERIOD

Client signature _____ Date_____

FOLLOW-UP CONSULTATION # 4

Client's name	Address
Therapist's name	Date

STATE OF HEALTH SINCE THE LAST APPOINTMENT

Have the symptoms presented last time improved/ got worse? How have they changed?	
Digestion	
Elimination	
Sleep	
Stress	
Energy levels/ fatigue	
General state of health	
Mental state	

Have you followed the recommendations and agreed diet plan?
_____
_____
_____

What do you think helped you most?
_____
_____
_____

What didn't help?
_____
_____
_____

What changes would you like to make to your diet?
_____
_____
_____

What changes would you like to make to your lifestyle?
_____
_____
_____

AGREED PLAN FOR THE NEXT AGREED PERIOD

```
┌─────────────────────────────────────────────────────────────┐
│                                                             │
│                                                             │
│                                                             │
│                                                             │
│                                                             │
└─────────────────────────────────────────────────────────────┘
```

Client signature _____ Date_____

AGREED WEEKLY DIET & HEALTH MANAGEMENT PLAN

Monday

Breakfast	Lunch
Dinner	Snacks
Water	Sleep
Exercise	Relaxation routines
Fasting periods (if any)	Supplements

Tuesday

Breakfast	Lunch
Dinner	Snacks
Water	Sleep
Exercise	Relaxation routines
Fasting periods (if any)	Supplements

Wednesday

Breakfast	Lunch
Dinner	Snacks
Water	Sleep
Exercise	Relaxation routines
Fasting periods (if any)	Supplements

Thursday

Breakfast	Lunch
Dinner	Snacks
Water	Sleep
Exercise	Relaxation routines
Fasting periods (if any)	Supplements

Friday

Breakfast	Lunch
Dinner	Snacks
Water	Sleep
Exercise	Relaxation routines
Fasting periods (if any)	Supplements

Saturday

Breakfast	Lunch
Dinner	Snacks
Water	Sleep
Exercise	Relaxation routines
Fasting periods (if any)	Supplements

Sunday

Breakfast	Lunch
Dinner	Snacks
Water	Sleep
Exercise	Relaxation routines
Fasting periods (if any)	Supplements

Weekly Results & Observations

Therapist's Notes

Notes

Notes

Notes

Notes

Notes

Notes

Notes

Notes

Notes

Notes

Notes

Printed in Great Britain
by Amazon